I'm A Little Yogi

YOGA FOR CHILDREN

For my niece Aaliyah Keana

AuthorHouse™
1663 Liberty Drive
Bloomington, IN 47403
www.authorhouse.com
Phone: 1-800-839-8640

Published by AuthorHouse 04/16/2013

ISBN: 978-1-4817-3708-1 (sc)
978-1-4817-3709-8 (e)

Library of Congress Control Number: 2013906547

This book is printed on acid-free paper.

authorHOUSE®

What is Yoga?

Yoga is a Sanskrit word meaning to yoke or to unite. It is a combination of physical practice (poses), breathing, and concentration (which leads to meditation). Practicing yoga happens when you bring your body and mind together and become present in the moment.

A little yogi is a young person practicing yoga.

The Meaning of Namaste

Namaste means "I bow to you" or "salutations to you," an English equivalent is saying "greetings" or "good day". The gesture of placing the hands together, bowing down and saying "Namaste" is a symbol of gratitude and respect. It can be used universally while meeting another person.

Benefits of practicing yoga with your Little Yogi

~ Better concentration
~ Better body awareness
~ Strengthens the body
~ Improves coordination

~ Increases creativity
~ Better listening skills
~ Increases flexibility

~ Increases self-esteem
~ Family bonding
~ Relaxing

Suggestions to Readers

You can read this book to your little yogi while acting out each pose. You can chose to read from beginning to end then re-read the story or read the same page twice to ensure you stretch and strengthen both sides of the body.

Yoga with children is meant to be fun and playful. Practice with your child so that he or she can follow you.

Pose Instructions

Mountain Pose: Stand tall with both feet planted on the ground. Relax your arms by your sides and open your chest.

Star Pose: Standing tall, spread your feet as wide as you can and stretch your arms out to shoulder height.

Triangle Pose: Stand tall with your feet as wide as you can. Turn your right foot out and stretch your arms up to your shoulders. Turn your head to look over your right hand and bend your torso over your right leg. Look down to your big toe or up to your thumb. Repeat on your left side.

Airplane Pose: Stand with feet hip width apart, take a big step with your right foot and stretch your arms out to your sides. Place your weight on your right foot and lift your left leg straight behind you as you lower your torso until your body is parallel to the floor. Repeat on your left leg.

Downward Dog Pose: From your hands and knees, tuck your toes under and press them into the floor. Lift your hips and bottom as high as your can while pushing the floor away with your hands and bringing your heels close to the floor.

Easy Pose (Seated): Sit tall with your sits bones on the floor and cross your legs. Repeat with the other leg in front.

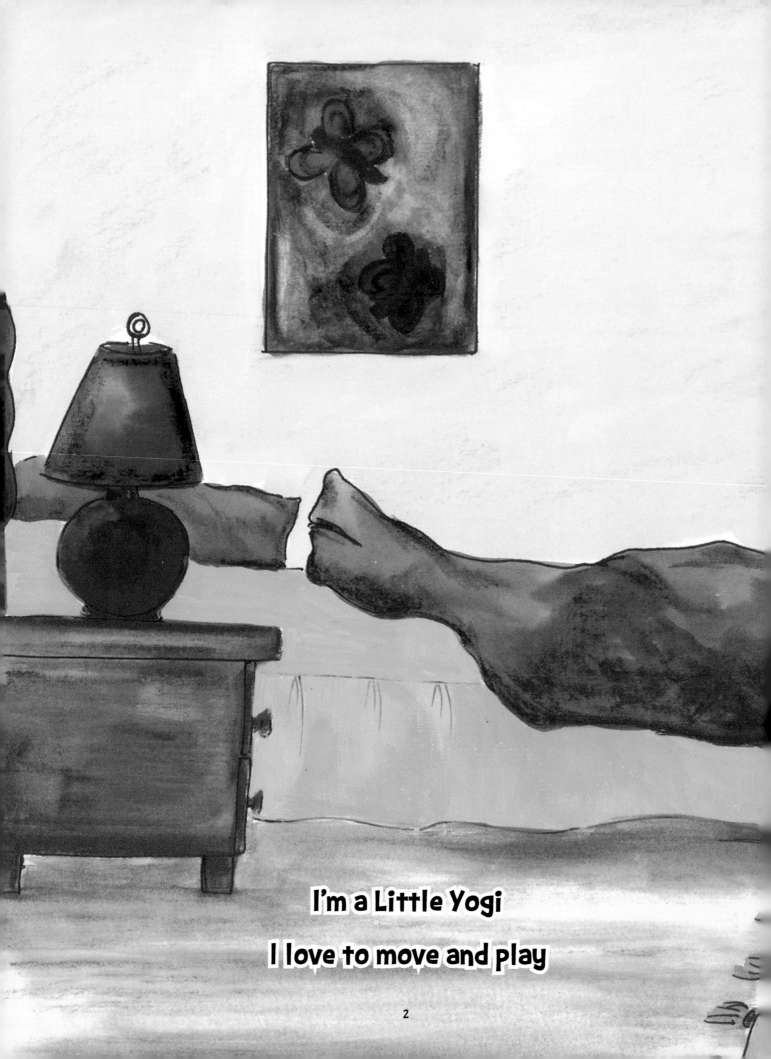

I'm a Little Yogi
I love to move and play

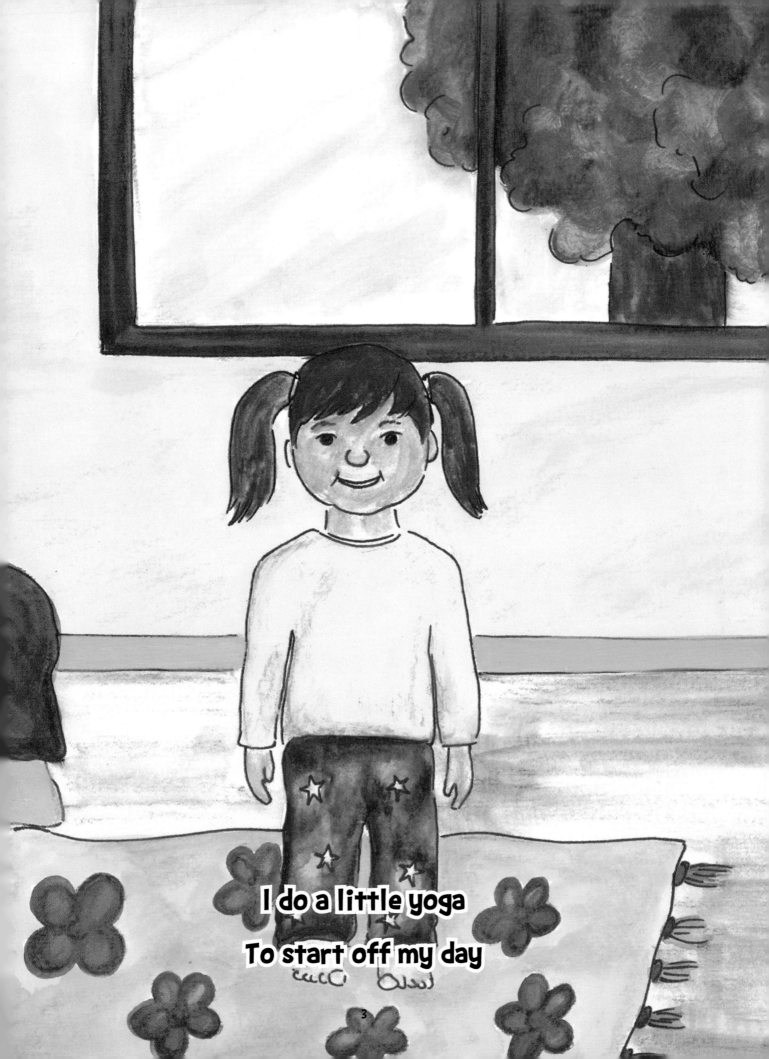

I do a little yoga
To start off my day

3

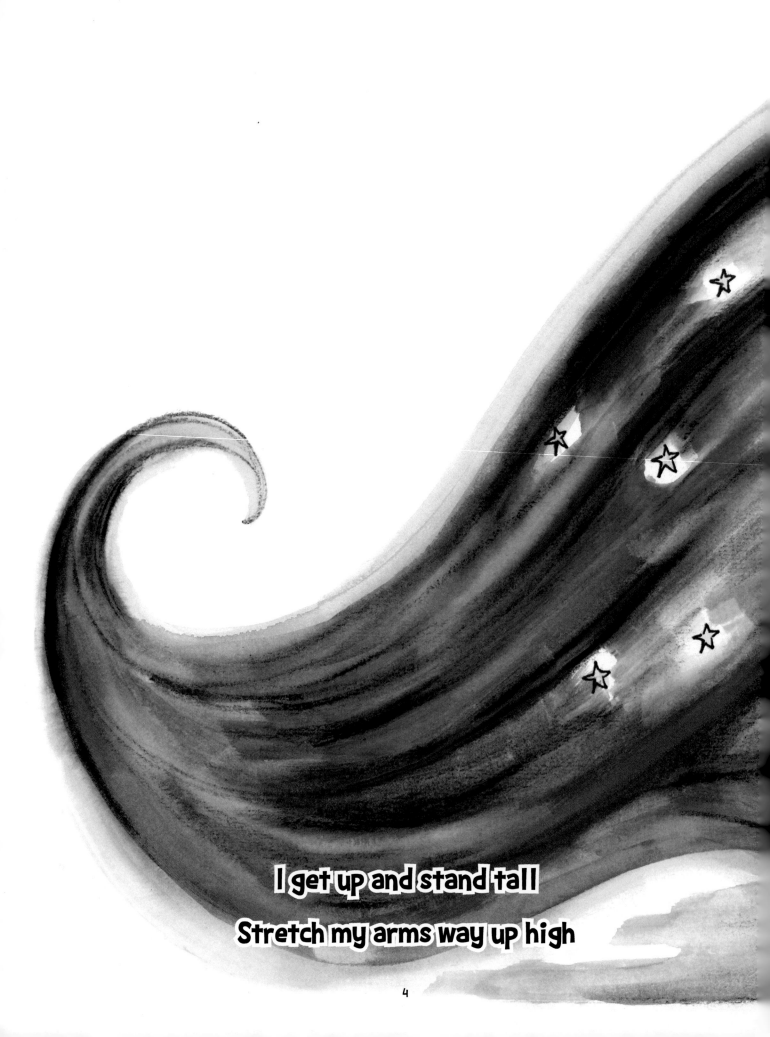

I get up and stand tall
Stretch my arms way up high

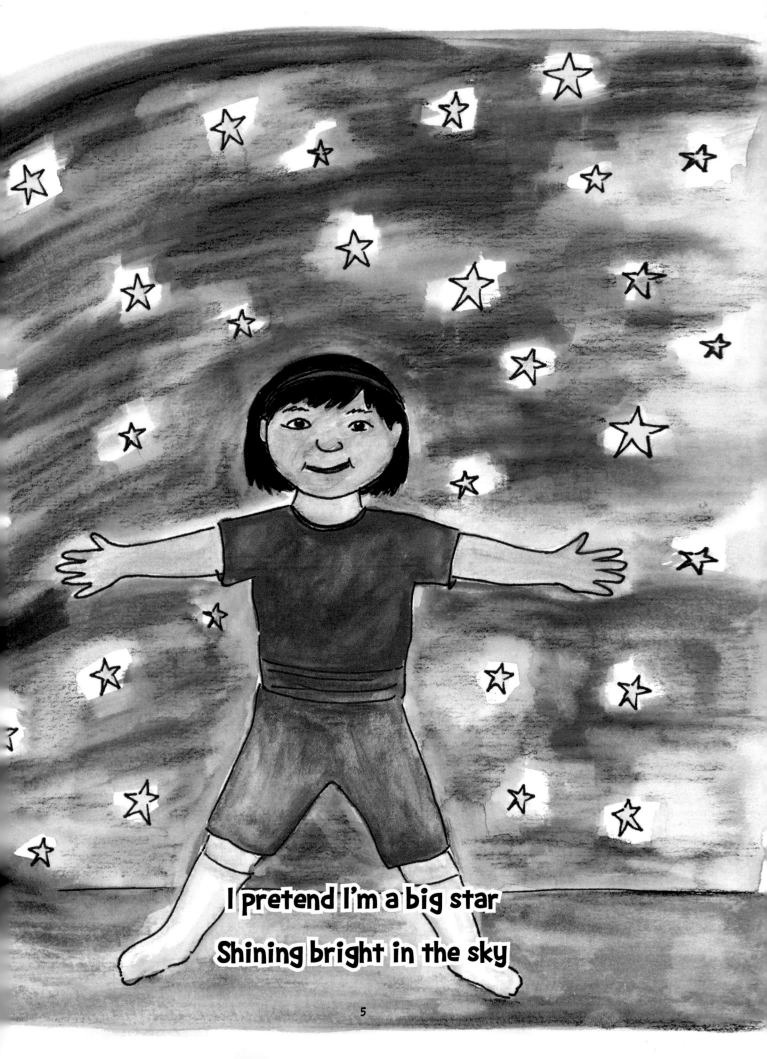

I pretend I'm a big star

Shining bright in the sky

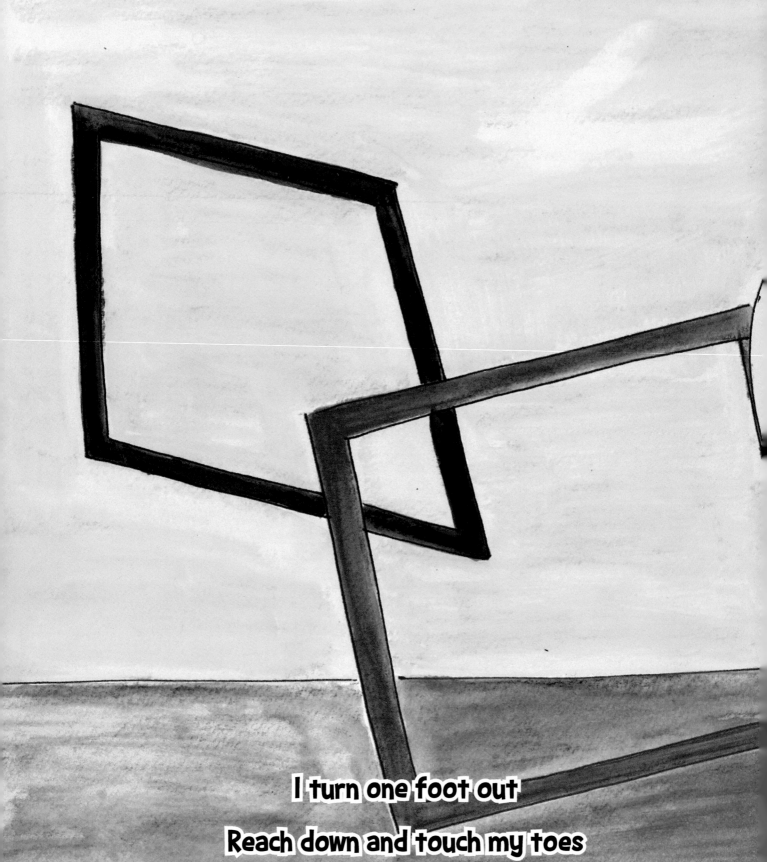

I turn one foot out

Reach down and touch my toes

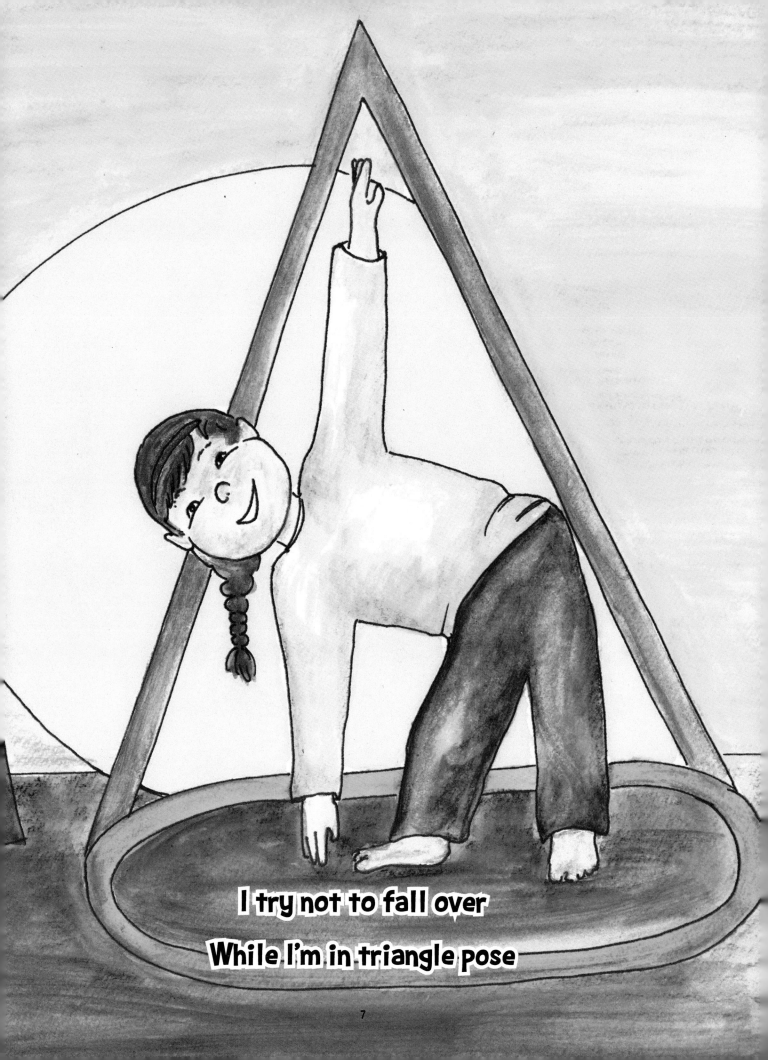

I try not to fall over
While I'm in triangle pose

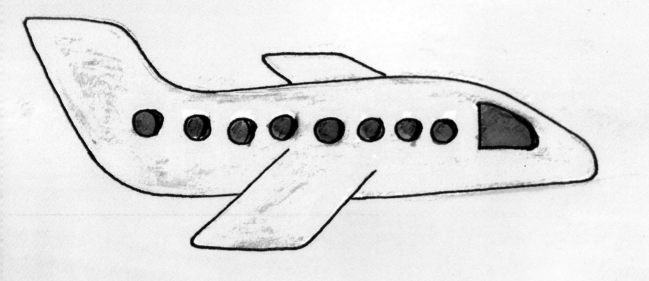

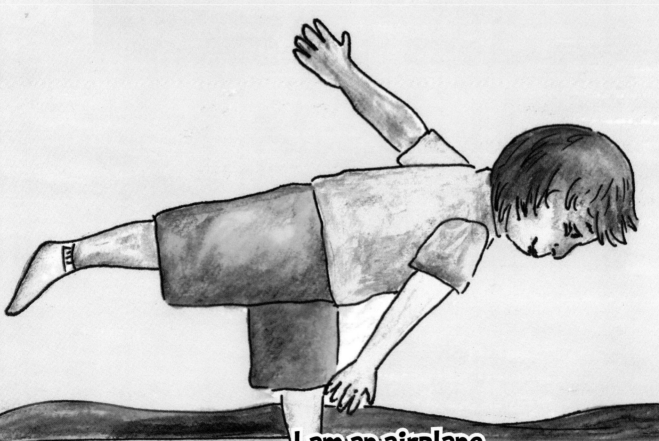

I am an airplane

Flying to places all around

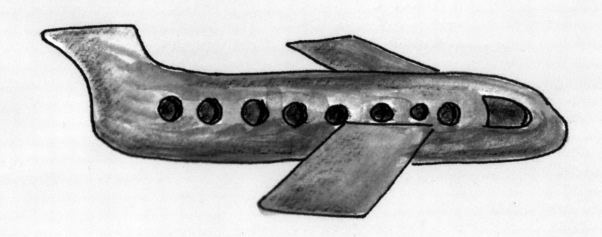
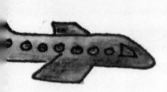

Standing on one foot, arms out

Looking down on the ground

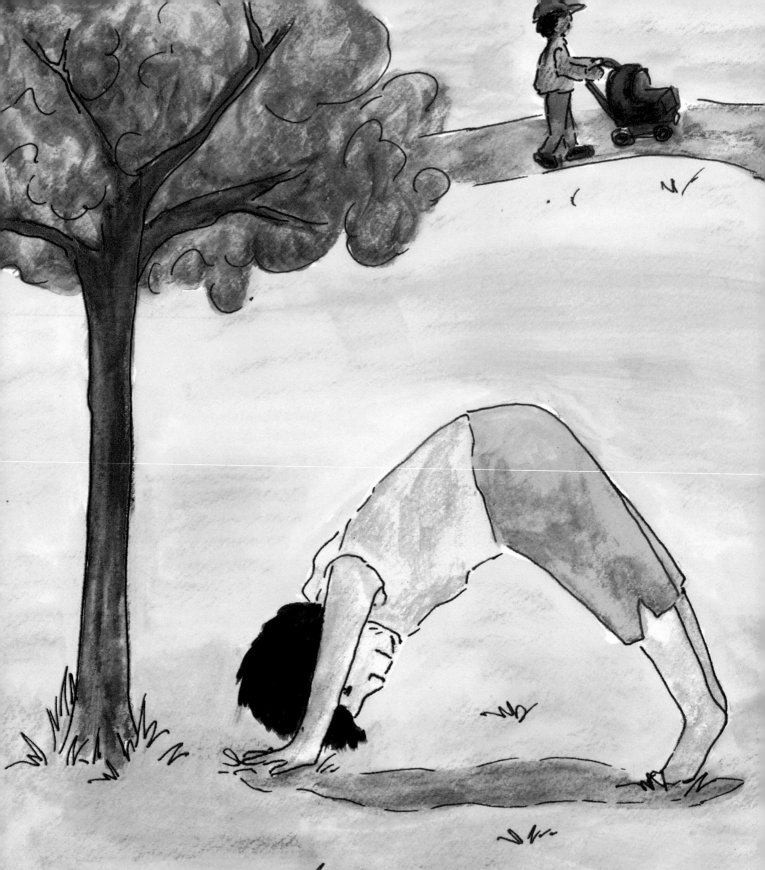

With my hands on the floor

And bottom way up high

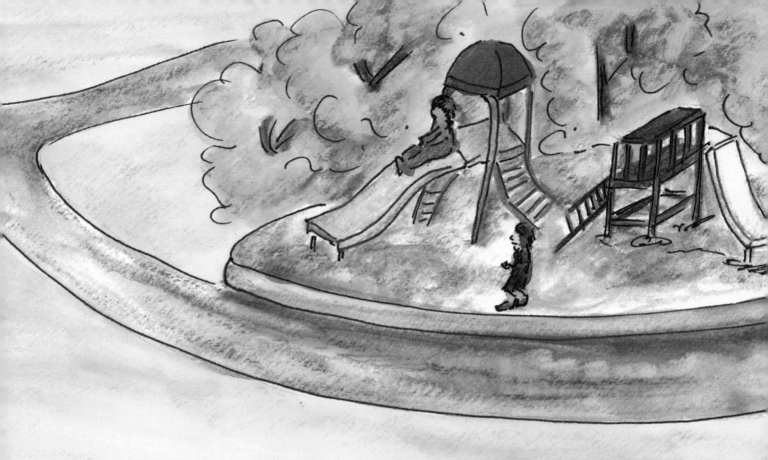

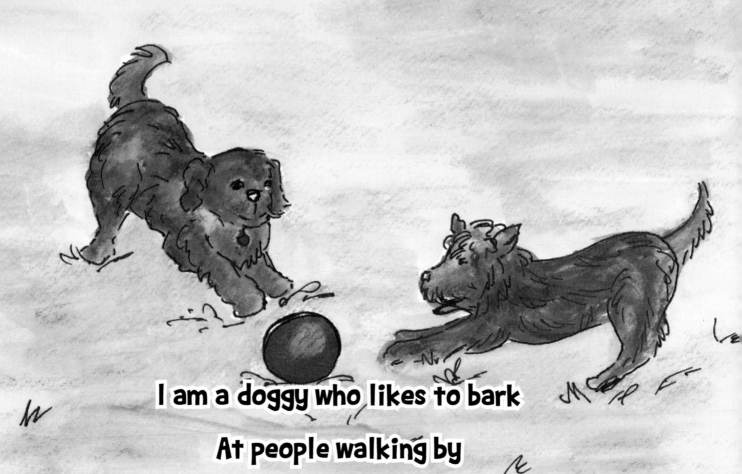

I am a doggy who likes to bark
At people walking by

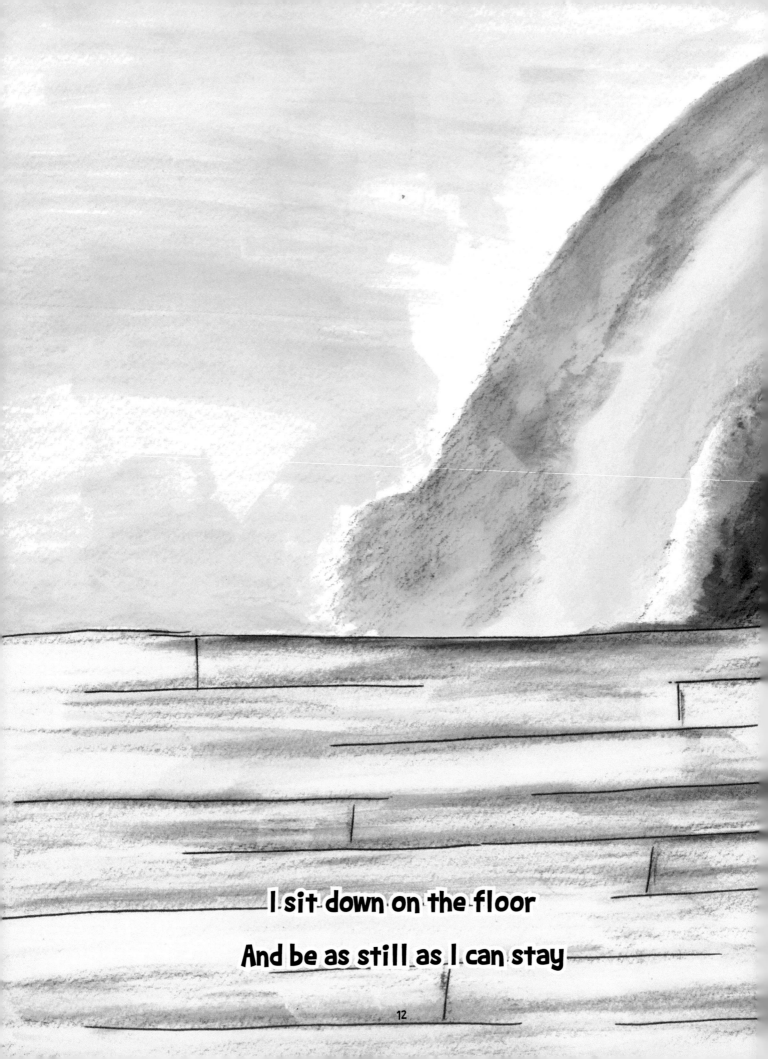

I sit down on the floor
And be as still as I can stay

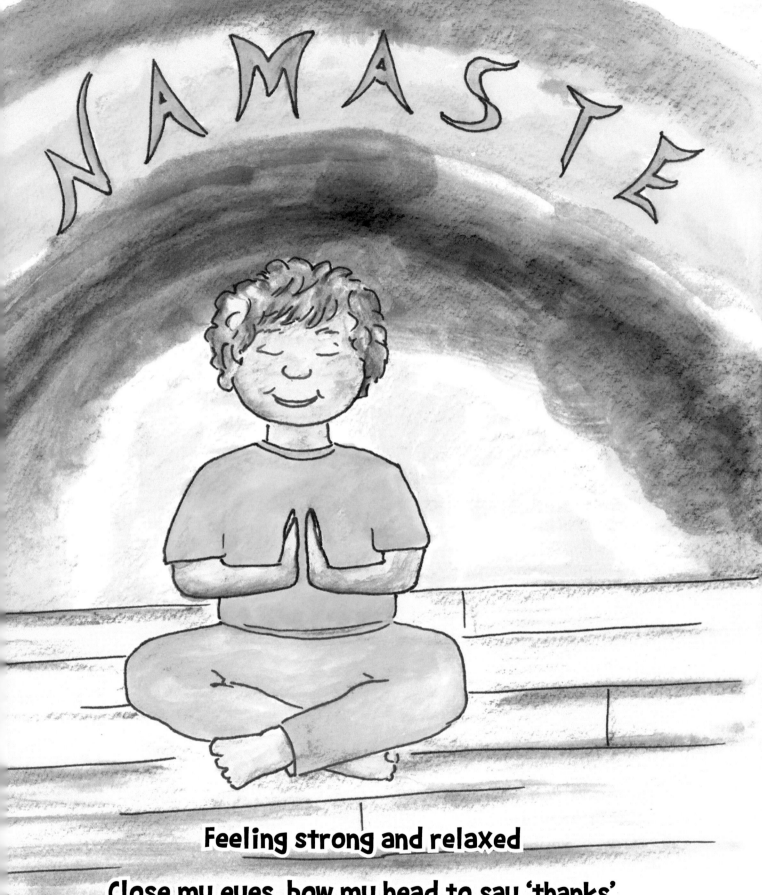

NAMASTE

Feeling strong and relaxed

Close my eyes, bow my head to say 'thanks'

Namaste, Namaste, Namaste!

CPSIA information can be obtained
at www.ICGtesting.com
Printed in the USA
LVIC041329080513
332870LV00001B

9 781481 737081